NATURAL AND PERMANENT SOLUTIONS FOR VAGINAL HEALTH

Managing Odor And Discharge

Dr. Arthur Myles

TABLE OF CONTENTS

INTRODUCTION

Vaginal health is a cornerstone of a woman's overall well-being. A healthy vagina naturally maintains its balance with the help of good bacteria, an acidic pH, and regular secretions that cleanse and protect the area. However, various factors like lifestyle choices, hormonal changes, and external irritants can disrupt this balance, leading to issues such as unpleasant odor and abnormal discharge.

Understanding what's normal and what's not is the first step toward addressing these concerns. While mild odor and clear or white discharge are natural, changes in color, consistency, or a strong, unpleasant smell may indicate an underlying issue that requires attention.

This guide focuses on natural and permanent solutions to promote vaginal health, manage odor, and regulate discharge. By integrating proper hygiene, dietary changes, natural remedies, and lifestyle adjustments, women can support their vaginal health in a holistic and lasting way.

Whether you're looking to prevent recurring problems or enhance your current routine, the solutions in this guide aim to empower you with safe, effective, and sustainable practices. Remember, it's always important to seek professional advice if symptoms persist or cause discomfort.

CHAPTER 1
Maintaining Proper Hygiene

Proper hygiene is essential for maintaining vaginal health and preventing issues such as odor, abnormal discharge, and infections. The vaginal area is self-cleaning, and a balanced approach to hygiene is often more effective than over-cleaning or using harsh products. Here are practical tips for maintaining optimal hygiene:

Gentle Cleansing Practices

Wash with Warm Water: Use lukewarm water to clean the external genital area daily. Avoid scrubbing, which can cause irritation.

Choose Mild, Fragrance-Free Products: Opt for gentle, pH-balanced, fragrance-free soaps or cleansers specifically formulated for the vaginal area. Harsh soaps can disrupt the natural bacterial balance.

Avoid Douching: Douching can upset the natural flora and pH of the vagina, increasing the risk of infections such as bacterial vaginosis.

Wear Breathable Underwear

Choose Cotton: Cotton underwear allows air circulation and helps wick away moisture, reducing the risk of bacterial and fungal growth.

Avoid Tight Clothing: Tight pants or synthetic fabrics can trap heat and moisture, creating an environment conducive to infections.

Practice Proper Wiping Techniques
Front to Back: Always wipe from front to back after using the toilet to prevent the transfer of bacteria from the anus to the vaginal area.
Gentle Patting: Use soft tissue or a clean cloth to gently pat the area dry after washing or wiping.

Change Pads and Tampons Regularly
During Menstruation: Change tampons or pads every 4-6 hours, or more frequently if needed, to prevent irritation and infections.
Opt for Unscented Products: Use unscented pads and tampons to avoid exposure to unnecessary chemicals or fragrances.

Manage Moisture
Avoid Prolonged Wetness: Change out of wet swimsuits or sweaty workout clothes as soon as possible to reduce moisture that can encourage bacterial or fungal growth.
Use Panty Liners Sparingly: If you use panty liners, opt for unscented and breathable ones, and change them frequently to keep the area dry.

By adopting these simple yet effective hygiene practices, you can protect your vaginal health and reduce the risk of discomfort, odor, and infections.

Regular attention to these habits supports the body's natural ability to maintain balance and cleanliness.

CHAPTER 2
Diet and Hydration

A healthy diet and proper hydration play a crucial role in supporting vaginal health. The food and drinks you consume can impact your body's natural balance, immune system, and pH levels, which are essential for preventing odor and abnormal discharge. Incorporating the right nutrients and staying hydrated can help maintain the health of the vaginal flora and overall well-being.

Probiotic-Rich Foods

Why They Help: Probiotics contain beneficial bacteria (Lactobacillus) that support a healthy vaginal microbiome by maintaining the right pH and preventing overgrowth of harmful bacteria.

What to Include:
Yogurt (with live, active cultures)
Kefir
Sauerkraut
Kimchi
Miso
Fermented pickles
Probiotic supplements (consult with a healthcare provider for recommendations)

Hydration

Why It Matters: Proper hydration aids in flushing out toxins and supports natural vaginal lubrication, reducing dryness and discomfort.
Tips for Staying Hydrated:
Drink at least 8 glasses (2 liters) of water daily, more if you're physically active or in hot weather.
Consume water-rich foods like cucumbers, watermelons, and oranges.

Cranberry Juice

Why It's Beneficial: Unsweetened cranberry juice is known for its ability to prevent urinary tract infections (UTIs) by preventing bacteria from adhering to the bladder walls.
How to Use It: Drink a small glass of pure, unsweetened cranberry juice daily or take cranberry supplements as a preventative measure.

Foods Rich in Antioxidants

Why They Help: Antioxidants reduce inflammation and boost immunity, helping the body fight infections and maintain a healthy vaginal environment.
What to Include:
Blueberries, strawberries, and other berries
Dark leafy greens like spinach and kale
Nuts and seeds (e.g., almonds, walnuts, sunflower seeds)
Green tea

Balanced Nutrition

General Principles: A diet rich in essential nutrients promotes overall health and hormonal balance. Focus on the following:
Fruits and Vegetables: Provide vitamins, minerals, and fiber for gut and vaginal health.
Whole Grains: Brown rice, quinoa, and oats support digestion and reduce inflammation.
Lean Proteins: Fish, chicken, eggs, and plant-based proteins help with tissue repair and immune health.
Healthy Fats: Include sources like avocados, olive oil, and fatty fish for hormonal balance and cellular health.

Minimize Sugar and Processed Foods

Why to Avoid Them: High sugar intake can promote yeast overgrowth, leading to infections such as candidiasis. Processed foods often contain preservatives and additives that can disrupt the body's balance.

What to Reduce:
Sugary snacks and beverages
Processed and fried foods
Refined carbohydrates like white bread and pastries

By focusing on a nutrient-rich, balanced diet and staying hydrated, you can enhance your vaginal health and overall vitality. These dietary adjustments not only address immediate concerns like odor and discharge but also create a foundation for long-term wellness.

CHAPTER 3
Natural Remedies

Incorporating natural remedies into your routine can be an effective and gentle way to support vaginal health, manage odor, and regulate discharge. These remedies leverage the antimicrobial, antifungal, and balancing properties of natural ingredients to address common concerns without harsh chemicals.

Apple Cider Vinegar (ACV) Baths
Benefits: Apple cider vinegar helps restore the natural pH balance of the vagina and has mild antibacterial and antifungal properties.

How to Use:
Add 1-2 cups of raw, unfiltered apple cider vinegar to a warm bath.
Soak for 15-20 minutes, 2-3 times per week.
Note: Avoid direct application inside the vagina, as it can be too strong and cause irritation.

Tea Tree Oil
Benefits: Tea tree oil has potent antimicrobial and antifungal properties, making it effective against infections like yeast and bacterial vaginosis.

How to Use:
Dilute 3-5 drops of tea tree oil In 1 tablespoon of a carrier oil (e.g., coconut oil).

Apply externally to the vaginal area.
Alternatively, use tea tree oil suppositories designed for vaginal use.
Caution: Always perform a patch test to ensure you're not allergic, and never use undiluted tea tree oil.

Coconut Oil

Benefits: Coconut oil is a natural moisturizer with antifungal properties, helpful for managing yeast infections and soothing irritation.

How to Use:
Use organic, cold-pressed coconut oil.
Apply a small amount externally or use as a base for mixing with essential oils like tea tree.

Garlic

Benefits: Garlic contains allicin, a compound with antimicrobial and antifungal effects, which may help fight infections.

How to Use:
Consume 1-2 raw cloves daily or include garlic in your meals.
For targeted use, consult a healthcare provider about using garlic supplements.
Caution: Avoid direct application of garlic to the vaginal area, as it may cause irritation.

Plain Yogurt

Benefits: Plain, unsweetened yogurt with live cultures can help replenish healthy bacteria in the vagina.

How to Use:
Eat yogurt regularly to support overall gut and vaginal health.
For external use, apply a small amount of yogurt directly to the vulva or use as a vaginal suppository.
Leave it on for 20-30 minutes, then rinse with warm water.

Aloe Vera
Benefits: Aloe vera soothes irritation, reduces inflammation, and helps maintain hydration.

How to Use:
Use pure aloe vera gel (without added chemicals or fragrances).
Apply externally to soothe irritation and dryness.

Fenugreek Seeds
Benefits: Fenugreek helps regulate hormones, supporting a healthy menstrual cycle and vaginal health.

How to Use:
Soak 1-2 tablespoons of fenugreek seeds in water overnight, then drink the strained water on an empty stomach.
Alternatively, consume fenugreek tea or supplements.

Boric Acid Suppositories

Benefits: Boric acid helps restore pH balance and is effective against recurring infections like bacterial vaginosis and yeast infections.

How to Use:
Use boric acid suppositories as directed by a healthcare provider.
Insert into the vagina once daily, typically for 7-14 days.
Caution: Never ingest boric acid, and avoid use during pregnancy unless prescribed by a doctor.

Tips for Using Natural Remedies Safely

Always test remedies on a small patch of skin first to check for allergic reactions.
Use remedies consistently but avoid overuse, which can disrupt natural balance.
Consult a healthcare provider if symptoms persist or worsen, as some conditions may require medical treatment.

These natural remedies can complement your efforts to maintain vaginal health, offering safe and effective solutions for common concerns.

CHAPTER 4
Lifestyle Adjustments

In addition to proper hygiene, diet, and natural remedies, lifestyle factors play a significant role in maintaining optimal vaginal health. Making a few key lifestyle adjustments can help balance hormones, boost the immune system, and prevent recurring issues like odor, discharge, and infections.

Stress Management

Why It Helps: Chronic stress can disrupt hormonal balance, weaken the immune system, and increase the risk of infections, including yeast infections.

How to Manage Stress:
Practice Mindfulness: Meditation, deep breathing exercises, or yoga can help reduce stress levels.
Engage in Relaxing Hobbies: Reading, crafting, or spending time outdoors can help unwind and lower stress.
Set Boundaries: Prioritize self-care and avoid overcommitting to reduce stress from work or personal life.

Regular Physical Activity

Why It Helps: Regular exercise improves blood circulation, supports hormone regulation, strengthens the immune system, and promotes overall vaginal health.

How to Stay Active:
Engage in at least 150 minutes of moderate exercise per week, such as walking, cycling, or swimming.
Practice strength training or yoga to improve pelvic floor health and prevent urinary incontinence.
Avoid excessive use of tight workout clothing to reduce the risk of irritation and moisture buildup.

Adequate Sleep
Why It Helps: Sufficient sleep allows the body to repair itself, regulate hormones, and support the immune system, all of which are essential for vaginal health.

How to Improve Sleep:
Aim for 7-9 hours of sleep each night.
Establish a consistent bedtime routine and avoid using screens at least 30 minutes before sleep.
Create a calm and dark sleep environment to promote restful sleep.

Maintain a Healthy Weight
Why It Helps: Being overweight can disrupt hormonal balance and increase the likelihood of infections like yeast infections. Maintaining a healthy weight supports overall reproductive and vaginal health.

How to Manage Weight:
Follow a balanced, nutrient-rich diet and incorporate regular physical activity into your daily routine.

Practice portion control and eat mindfully to avoid overeating.

Smoking Cessation
Why It Helps: Smoking weakens the immune system and can increase the risk of infections, including bacterial vaginosis. It can also negatively affect circulation and vaginal lubrication.

How to Quit:
Seek professional help if needed, such as counseling, nicotine replacement therapy, or support groups.
Engage in activities that reduce cravings, such as walking, chewing gum, or practicing deep breathing exercises.

Stay Hydrated
Why It Helps: Hydration supports the body's natural detox processes, helps flush out toxins, and supports vaginal lubrication.

How to Stay Hydrated:
Aim to drink at least 8 glasses (2 liters) of water per day, more if you exercise or live in a hot climate.
Include water-rich foods in your diet, such as cucumbers, watermelon, and oranges.

Avoid Excessive Use of Scented Products
Why It Helps: Scented products like sprays, douches, or powders can disrupt the natural balance of bacteria

and pH in the vagina, leading to irritation and infections.

What to Avoid:
Scented sanitary pads, tampons, or panty liners.
Vaginal deodorants or sprays.
Bubble baths or heavily perfumed soaps.
What to Use Instead: Stick to unscented, hypoallergenic, and pH-balanced products.

Maintain Good Sexual Health Practices
Why It Helps: Safe sexual practices protect against sexually transmitted infections (STIs), which can affect vaginal health.

How to Stay Safe:
Use condoms or dental dams during sexual activity to reduce the risk of STIs.
Urinate after sex to flush out any bacteria that may have entered the urethra.
Ensure open communication with your partner about sexual health and hygiene.

By incorporating these lifestyle adjustments, you can improve your overall health and create an environment that supports vaginal well-being. These changes may seem small but can have a lasting impact on your health, helping you prevent discomfort and maintain a balanced, healthy vaginal ecosystem.

CHAPTER 5
Avoiding Irritants

Certain products and habits can introduce chemicals or substances that disrupt the natural balance of the vaginal area, leading to irritation, infections, or discomfort. Identifying and avoiding these irritants is crucial for maintaining vaginal health and preventing issues like abnormal discharge, odor, or itching. Here are some common irritants to avoid:

Scented Products

Why to Avoid: Scented products, including vaginal sprays, deodorants, and scented tampons or pads, contain chemicals that can irritate sensitive skin and disrupt the natural pH balance of the vagina.

What to Avoid:
Scented sanitary products (pads, tampons, panty liners)
Vaginal sprays or douches .
Perfumed soaps and body washes
Alternatives: Choose unscented, hypoallergenic products specifically designed for sensitive skin or the vaginal area.

Douching

Why to Avoid: Douching, or the practice of rinsing the vagina with water or solutions (often containing fragrances or chemicals), can disrupt the natural balance of bacteria and pH, leading to infections like bacterial vaginosis and yeast infections.

What to Avoid:
Commercial douches or any type of internal washing product.
Alternatives: The vagina is self-cleaning, so avoid inserting anything into it. Instead, wash the external genital area with warm water and mild, fragrance-free soap.

Tight Clothing and Synthetic Fabrics
Why to Avoid: Tight clothing, especially synthetic fabrics like nylon or polyester, can trap moisture and heat, creating an environment where bacteria and fungi can thrive. This can lead to conditions like yeast infections and irritation.

What to Avoid:
Tight-fitting pants, leggings, or underwear made of synthetic fabrics.
Alternatives: Choose loose-fitting, breathable clothing and underwear made of natural fabrics like cotton that allow airflow and wick moisture away from the body.

Harsh Chemical Soaps or Body Washes
Why to Avoid: Soaps and body washes with strong fragrances or harsh chemicals can irritate the sensitive skin of the genital area, leading to dryness, itching, or an imbalance in the vaginal microbiome.

What to Avoid:
Soaps with artificial fragrances, alcohol, or strong chemicals.
Alternatives: Use mild, fragrance-free soaps or cleansers specifically designed for the genital area. Consider gentle, pH-balanced products to preserve the natural acidity of the vagina.

Overuse of Antibacterial Products
Why to Avoid: While antibacterial products are designed to eliminate harmful bacteria, they can also kill the beneficial bacteria that maintain vaginal health, leading to an imbalance that may cause infections.

What to Avoid:
Antibacterial wipes, soaps, or gels applied to the genital area.
Alternatives: Stick to gentle, non-antibacterial products for regular hygiene and allow the body's natural defenses to manage bacteria.

Perfumed Toilet Paper or Wipes
Why to Avoid: Toilet paper or wipes with fragrances or harsh chemicals can cause irritation, especially for those with sensitive skin or prone to allergies.

What to Avoid:
Scented toilet paper or wipes.

Alternatives: Use unscented, hypoallergenic toilet paper, or consider using water and soft cloths for gentle cleaning.

Prolonged Use of Panty Liners

Why to Avoid: While panty liners are designed to absorb moisture, prolonged use can trap sweat and bacteria, potentially leading to irritation, yeast infections, or bacterial infections.

What to Avoid:
Daily use of panty liners, especially scented ones.
Alternatives: Use panty liners only when necessary and choose breathable, unscented options. Be sure to change them frequently to maintain dryness and comfort.

Use of Certain Medications

Why to Avoid: Some medications, like antibiotics, can disrupt the natural balance of vaginal flora by killing beneficial bacteria. This can lead to yeast infections or other imbalances.

What to Avoid:
Long-term or frequent use of antibiotics without probiotics.
Alternatives: Consult your healthcare provider about taking probiotics when using antibiotics, or inquire about alternatives for managing conditions that may require long-term medication use.

Scented or Harsh Laundry Detergents
Why to Avoid: Laundry detergents with strong fragrances or harsh chemicals can leave residues on clothing, including underwear, which may irritate the vaginal area.

What to Avoid:
Scented laundry detergents, fabric softeners, or dryer sheets.
Alternatives: Use unscented, hypoallergenic detergents and avoid fabric softeners or dryer sheets that contain fragrances.

General Tips for Avoiding Irritants
Wear cotton underwear and avoid tight-fitting clothes that trap moisture.
Choose natural or hypoallergenic products for personal care, and always opt for unscented versions when possible.
Give your skin time to breathe by changing out of sweaty clothes quickly and avoiding prolonged use of panty liners.
Be mindful of your laundry products and opt for detergents free from fragrances and harsh chemicals.

By avoiding these common irritants, you can help maintain the natural balance of your vaginal flora, prevent discomfort, and reduce the risk of infections and other vaginal health issues.

CHAPTER 6
Promoting Natural pH Balance

The vaginal pH plays a crucial role in maintaining a healthy balance of bacteria and yeast. A normal vaginal pH is slightly acidic, typically between 3.8 and 4.5, which helps prevent the overgrowth of harmful organisms and supports the growth of beneficial bacteria like Lactobacillus. When the pH balance is disrupted, it can lead to infections, odors, and discomfort. Promoting and maintaining a natural pH balance is key to vaginal health. Here are several strategies to help maintain or restore the vaginal pH balance:

Avoid Harsh Chemicals and Fragrances

Why It Helps: Harsh chemicals and fragrances in soaps, lotions, and other personal care products can irritate the sensitive skin of the genital area and disrupt the natural acidic environment of the vagina.

How to Promote Balance:
Use mild, unscented, pH-balanced products designed for the genital area.
Avoid douching or using vaginal sprays, as they can disturb the pH and lead to infections.
Stick to products that are free of alcohol, fragrances, or strong chemicals.

Maintain Proper Hygiene Without Over-Cleansing

Why It Helps: Over-washing or using strong soaps can strip the vagina of its natural oils and healthy bacteria, upsetting the pH balance. However, inadequate hygiene can also lead to bacterial growth and infections.

How to Promote Balance:
Wash the external genital area with warm water and a gentle, pH-balanced cleanser.
Avoid internal washing (douching), as the vagina is self-cleaning.
Pat the area dry after bathing or showering to prevent moisture buildup, which can disrupt pH.

Probiotics for Vaginal Health
Why It Helps: Probiotics, particularly Lactobacillus species, play an important role in maintaining a healthy vaginal pH by producing lactic acid, which keeps the environment acidic and protects against harmful bacteria and yeast.

How to Promote Balance:
Eat probiotic-rich foods like yogurt, kefir, kimchi, sauerkraut, and miso.
Consider taking probiotic supplements, particularly those containing Lactobacillus strains, to support vaginal flora balance.
Consult with a healthcare provider for guidance on probiotic use.

Eat a pH-Balancing Diet

Why It Helps: The food you eat can influence your body's internal pH levels, including your vaginal pH. Eating a balanced diet with the right foods can support natural vaginal health.

How to Promote Balance:
Incorporate Acidic Foods: Foods like cranberries, citrus fruits, and fermented foods (yogurt, kimchi) help maintain a healthy acidic environment.
Avoid Excessive Sugar and Refined Carbs: High sugar intake can promote the growth of yeast, leading to infections and an imbalance in pH.
Drink Plenty of Water: Staying hydrated helps flush out toxins and supports overall vaginal health.
Increase Fiber: A fiber-rich diet supports gut health, which in turn helps balance the vaginal microbiome.

Hydration for pH Balance
Why It Helps: Proper hydration helps flush out toxins, maintain healthy mucus membranes, and promote natural lubrication. This also aids in maintaining a balanced pH in the vaginal area.

How to Promote Balance:
Aim to drink at least 8 glasses (2 liters) of water per day.
Include water-rich foods in your diet, such as cucumbers, watermelon, and celery.
Limit sugary drinks, which can contribute to yeast growth and imbalance.

Avoid Tight Clothing and Synthetic Fabrics
Why It Helps: Tight clothing, especially made of synthetic materials, can trap moisture and heat, creating an environment where bacteria and yeast thrive. This can lead to irritation and disrupt pH balance.

How to Promote Balance:
Wear breathable, cotton underwear that allows air circulation and prevents moisture buildup.
Avoid tight-fitting pants, leggings, or synthetic fabrics that can trap heat.
Change out of sweaty clothes quickly to reduce moisture exposure.

Regular Sexual Health Practices
Why It Helps: Unprotected sexual activity can introduce bacteria or pathogens that disrupt the vaginal pH.

How to Promote Balance:
Use condoms or dental dams to reduce the risk of introducing harmful bacteria during sex.
Urinate after sex to help flush out any bacteria that may have entered the urethra.
Maintain open communication with your partner about sexual health and hygiene.
If using lubricants, choose water-based, unscented options to prevent irritation.

Monitor Antibiotic Use

Why It Helps: While antibiotics are essential for treating bacterial infections, they can also disrupt the vaginal microbiome by killing beneficial bacteria, leading to yeast infections and pH imbalance.

How to Promote Balance:
Take antibiotics only when prescribed by a healthcare provider.
Consider taking a probiotic supplement during and after a course of antibiotics to help restore healthy bacteria.
Avoid self-diagnosing and self-medicating, especially with antibiotics.

Manage Hormonal Fluctuations
Why It Helps: Hormonal changes, particularly during menstruation, pregnancy, or menopause, can affect vaginal pH, leading to imbalances.

How to Promote Balance:
Stay active and manage stress levels to help regulate hormones.
If you're experiencing hormonal changes (e.g., during menopause), talk to your healthcare provider about ways to manage vaginal health, such as using vaginal moisturizers or hormone replacement therapy (HRT) if appropriate.

By following these practices, you can promote and maintain a healthy vaginal pH, reducing the risk of discomfort, infections, and imbalances. Taking a holistic approach to vaginal health—through diet, hydration, proper hygiene, and lifestyle—can help you support the body's natural mechanisms and keep your vaginal flora balanced.

CHAPTER 7
Regular Check-Ups

Regular check-ups are an essential part of maintaining overall health, including vaginal health. Routine visits to a healthcare provider help detect potential issues early, manage existing conditions, and ensure that your reproductive system is functioning properly. Regular gynecological exams are particularly important for women to monitor and maintain vaginal health, address concerns, and prevent future complications. Here's how regular check-ups play a key role in vaginal health:

Annual Gynecological Exams

Why They Help: Annual visits to a gynecologist ensure that your reproductive health is assessed regularly. These exams help identify any abnormalities, infections, or conditions that might affect the vagina, cervix, uterus, or ovaries.

What to Expect:

Pelvic Exam: A physical examination to check for abnormalities in the reproductive organs (vagina, cervix, uterus, ovaries).

Pap Smear (Cervical Screening): This test screens for abnormal cell changes in the cervix that could lead to cervical cancer. It's usually recommended every 3 years for women between the ages of 21 and 65.

Breast Exam: The doctor may check your breasts for lumps or signs of breast cancer.
STI Testing: If you are sexually active, your doctor may recommend screening for sexually transmitted infections (STIs), such as chlamydia, gonorrhea, or HIV, depending on your risk factors.

Addressing Symptoms Early
Why It Helps: If you experience symptoms such as unusual discharge, odor, itching, pain, or discomfort in the vaginal area, a gynecological check-up can help diagnose the cause and prevent further issues.

What to Do:
Be open with your doctor about any symptoms you are experiencing.
Mention changes in vaginal discharge (color, consistency, odor), discomfort during sex, or other concerns that may indicate infection or hormonal imbalance.
Early diagnosis of conditions like yeast infections, bacterial vaginosis, or even more serious concerns like fibroids or cysts can prevent complications down the line.

Hormonal Health Monitoring
Why It Helps: Hormonal fluctuations can affect vaginal health, leading to dryness, irritation, or changes in discharge. Regular check-ups can help manage hormonal health and prevent issues related to menstruation, pregnancy, or menopause.

What to Expect:
Hormonal health assessments may be part of your regular check-up, particularly if you're going through menopause or experiencing irregular periods.
Your doctor may offer guidance on managing symptoms like vaginal dryness or discomfort during sex, and may recommend hormone therapy, lubricants, or other solutions to improve your quality of life.

STI Screening and Sexual Health

Why It Helps: Regular screening for sexually transmitted infections (STIs) is important for preventing the spread of infections and maintaining vaginal health. Many STIs can go unnoticed because they don't always cause symptoms, making regular testing crucial.

What to Do:
If you're sexually active, especially with multiple partners, discuss STI testing with your healthcare provider.
Get tested for common STIs like chlamydia, gonorrhea, syphilis, and HIV, even if you don't have symptoms.
If you're at high risk or have a history of abnormal pap smears or HPV, your doctor may recommend more frequent screenings.

Managing and Preventing Infections

Why It Helps: Frequent or recurring infections (e.g., yeast infections, bacterial vaginosis, urinary tract infections) can affect vaginal health. Regular visits can help identify the underlying cause of recurrent infections and determine an appropriate treatment plan.

What to Expect:
Your doctor will ask about your symptoms and may perform tests (e.g., urine tests, vaginal swabs) to determine the cause of infections.
If needed, they will provide treatment for infections and may offer lifestyle or dietary advice to help prevent future occurrences.
For recurring yeast infections or bacterial vaginosis, your doctor might suggest a longer-term treatment plan or additional diagnostic tests to rule out underlying conditions.

Cancer Screenings and Early Detection
Why It Helps: Early detection of cancers like cervical cancer, ovarian cancer, or vaginal cancer significantly improves treatment outcomes. Regular check-ups can help detect abnormal changes before they progress to more serious stages.

What to Expect:
Pap Smear: Regular pap smears screen for precancerous cells on the cervix that could develop into cervical cancer.

HPV Testing: Human papillomavirus (HPV) is a virus that can cause cervical cancer. Testing for HPV helps identify higher-risk strains.
Breast and Pelvic Exams: These exams can detect lumps, growths, or signs of cancer in the reproductive organs or breasts.
Ultrasounds or Blood Tests: Your doctor may recommend these if you experience symptoms that suggest ovarian or uterine issues.

Family Planning and Contraception
Why It Helps: If you're planning to have children or manage family size, discussing family planning options with your gynecologist is essential. Additionally, contraception can prevent unintended pregnancies and help manage menstrual cycles.

What to Expect:
Your doctor can help you explore various contraception options, including birth control pills, IUDs, implants, or natural methods.
If you're trying to conceive, your doctor can provide guidance on optimizing fertility and address any potential fertility issues.
If you are planning for pregnancy, your healthcare provider can recommend preconception care to ensure your body is ready for a healthy pregnancy.

Menopause and Post-Menopause Care
Why It Helps: As women approach menopause, hormonal shifts can cause various symptoms, such

as hot flashes, vaginal dryness, and mood swings.
Regular check-ups during and after menopause help
manage these symptoms and maintain vaginal
health.

What to Expect:
During menopause, your doctor can offer options for
managing symptoms like hormone replacement
therapy (HRT) or non-hormonal treatments for
vaginal dryness and discomfort.
Post-menopausal women should continue with
annual check-ups to monitor for signs of
osteoporosis, cardiovascular disease, and other
health concerns.

Benefits of Regular Check-Ups for Vaginal Health
Prevention: Regular visits help prevent infections,
cancers, and other issues before they become
serious.
Peace of Mind: Knowing that your vaginal health is
being monitored provides peace of mind and
encourages healthy habits.
Personalized Care: Your doctor can provide tailored
advice for managing symptoms, improving hygiene
practices, and maintaining overall well-being.

By scheduling and attending regular check-ups, you
empower yourself to stay proactive about your health,
detect potential problems early, and maintain the best
possible vaginal health. Don't hesitate to talk openly
with your healthcare provider about any concerns or

questions you may have—your reproductive health is
an essential part of your overall well-being.

CHAPTER 8
When to Seek Medical Attention

While many vaginal issues can be managed with proper hygiene and lifestyle changes, there are times when seeking medical attention is essential. Certain symptoms may indicate underlying conditions that require professional treatment or intervention. Knowing when to seek help can ensure early detection and appropriate care, reducing the risk of complications and promoting long-term vaginal health.

Unusual or Foul Odor

What to Look For:

A strong, foul-smelling odor, particularly one that is fishy or sour, can indicate bacterial vaginosis, a yeast infection, or other infections.

A musty odor that doesn't improve with regular hygiene may suggest a more serious underlying issue.

When to Seek Help: If the odor is persistent, unusually strong, or accompanied by other symptoms like itching, discomfort, or unusual discharge, it's important to consult a healthcare provider for diagnosis and treatment.

Unexplained Vaginal Discharge

What to Look For:

Discharge that is green, yellow, or gray in color, or has an unusual texture, may signal an infection.

A thick, white, cottage cheese-like discharge is common with a yeast infection, while watery discharge can be a symptom of bacterial vaginosis or other conditions.

If discharge changes dramatically in color, consistency, or volume, it is important to seek medical advice.

When to Seek Help: If the discharge is abnormal (e.g., foul-smelling, discolored, or accompanied by discomfort), seek a gynecologist's opinion for a proper diagnosis and treatment plan.

Pain or Discomfort During Sex

What to Look For:

Pain during intercourse can be a sign of vaginal dryness, infections, or more serious conditions like endometriosis, pelvic inflammatory disease (PID), or fibroids.

Discomfort may also occur due to hormonal imbalances, especially during menopause or after childbirth.

When to Seek Help: If pain during sex persists or worsens, or if it's accompanied by bleeding or other symptoms, consult a healthcare provider for further evaluation.

Itching, Burning, or Irritation

What to Look For:

Persistent itching, burning sensations, or irritation around the vaginal area could indicate a yeast infection, allergic reaction, or bacterial infection.

These symptoms, especially if they are severe or don't improve with over-the-counter treatments, should be addressed by a healthcare provider.

When to Seek Help: If the itching or burning is intense, doesn't go away after using over-the-counter remedies, or if it's accompanied by swelling, sores, or blisters, it's important to get medical advice.

Unexplained Bleeding

What to Look For:

Spotting or bleeding between periods, after sex, or after menopause can be a sign of an underlying condition such as an infection, hormonal imbalance, or more serious issues like cervical or uterine cancer. Postmenopausal bleeding is particularly concerning and should always be investigated.

When to Seek Help: If you experience any unexplained bleeding, especially between periods or after menopause, seek medical attention immediately for a thorough examination.

Pelvic or Abdominal Pain

What to Look For:

Persistent pelvic or lower abdominal pain can indicate conditions like pelvic inflammatory disease (PID), ovarian cysts, fibroids, or endometriosis.

Severe or sudden pain, particularly if it's accompanied by fever or nausea, should be addressed promptly.

When to Seek Help: If you experience severe or ongoing pelvic or abdominal pain, especially if it's accompanied by fever, vomiting, or abnormal vaginal discharge, you should consult a healthcare provider as soon as possible.

Frequent Urinary Tract Infections (UTIs)

What to Look For:

Symptoms of a UTI include a frequent urge to urinate, burning sensation during urination, cloudy or strong-smelling urine, and pelvic discomfort.

Recurrent UTIs may indicate an underlying issue that needs medical attention.

When to Seek Help: If you experience frequent UTIs or persistent symptoms despite treatment, it's important to consult with a doctor. They may recommend further tests or more targeted treatments to prevent future infections.

Swelling or Lumps in the Vaginal Area

What to Look For:

Swelling, lumps, or bumps near the vaginal opening could be cysts, abscesses, or warts, or they could indicate more serious conditions like genital herpes or cancer.

Painful or unusual lumps should always be checked by a healthcare professional.

When to Seek Help: If you find any unusual lumps or experience swelling in the vaginal area, particularly if they are painful or growing in size, it's important to seek medical attention for further evaluation.

Severe Vaginal Dryness
What to Look For:
Vaginal dryness is common during menopause, but it can also occur due to hormonal changes, medications, or breastfeeding.
If dryness is accompanied by pain during sex or frequent irritation, it may need medical treatment.
When to Seek Help: If vaginal dryness is affecting your daily life or causing discomfort, consult your doctor. They can recommend moisturizers, lubricants, or hormonal treatments to relieve symptoms.

Fever or Unexplained Symptoms
What to Look For:
If you have a fever along with vaginal pain, swelling, or unusual discharge, this may indicate a serious infection or other health concern that requires medical attention.
When to Seek Help: Any fever or unexplained symptoms, particularly when combined with pelvic pain, unusual discharge, or other vaginal health concerns, should be addressed by a healthcare provider.

It's important to listen to your body and seek medical help when you experience symptoms that are unusual, persistent, or cause concern. Early detection and treatment can prevent complications and ensure that any underlying conditions are properly addressed. If in doubt, always reach out to a healthcare professional to ensure that your vaginal health is in good condition. Regular check-ups and timely medical attention are key to maintaining long-term vaginal health and overall well-being.

CHAPTER 9
Conclusion

Vaginal health is a vital aspect of overall well-being, and maintaining it requires a holistic approach that combines self-care, lifestyle adjustments, and, when necessary, medical intervention. By taking proactive steps to care for your body—through proper hygiene, a balanced diet, natural remedies, and regular check-ups—you can foster long-term vaginal health and prevent many common issues. However, it's equally important to recognize when professional medical care is necessary to address more serious conditions or persistent symptoms.

The key to empowering long-term vaginal health lies in a balanced approach. This includes:

Maintaining Proper Hygiene: Gently cleanse the vaginal area, avoid harsh chemicals, and wear breathable clothing to support natural pH balance.

Supporting the Body Through Diet and Hydration: A nutrient-rich diet, adequate hydration, and probiotics play a significant role in maintaining vaginal health by supporting healthy bacteria and overall immunity.

Incorporating Natural Remedies: Herbal teas, essential oils, and other natural solutions can be used to promote vaginal comfort and balance, but they should complement, not replace, medical care.

Regular Check-Ups: Consistent visits to a healthcare provider ensure early detection of potential problems and allow for personalized guidance tailored to your unique needs.

When to Seek Medical Attention: Promptly addressing symptoms like unusual discharge, pain, itching, or discomfort ensures that underlying issues are diagnosed and treated effectively.

By combining natural approaches with medical guidance, you can create a balanced, sustainable routine that supports vaginal health. Always prioritize your comfort and well-being, and don't hesitate to seek professional help when needed. Empowering yourself with knowledge and care for your body allows you to enjoy a lifetime of optimal vaginal health and overall well-being.

Takeaways for Long-Term Vaginal Health:

Empathy and Self-Care: Take the time to care for your body through lifestyle choices, and listen to your body's signals.

Consistency and Balance: Regular check-ups, proper hygiene, a healthy diet, and hydration help maintain balance.

When in Doubt, Seek Help: Always consult a healthcare provider when symptoms are severe or persistent to ensure your health is protected.

Your vaginal health is part of your overall wellness journey. By combining the wisdom of natural remedies with medical expertise, you can achieve lasting health and confidence.

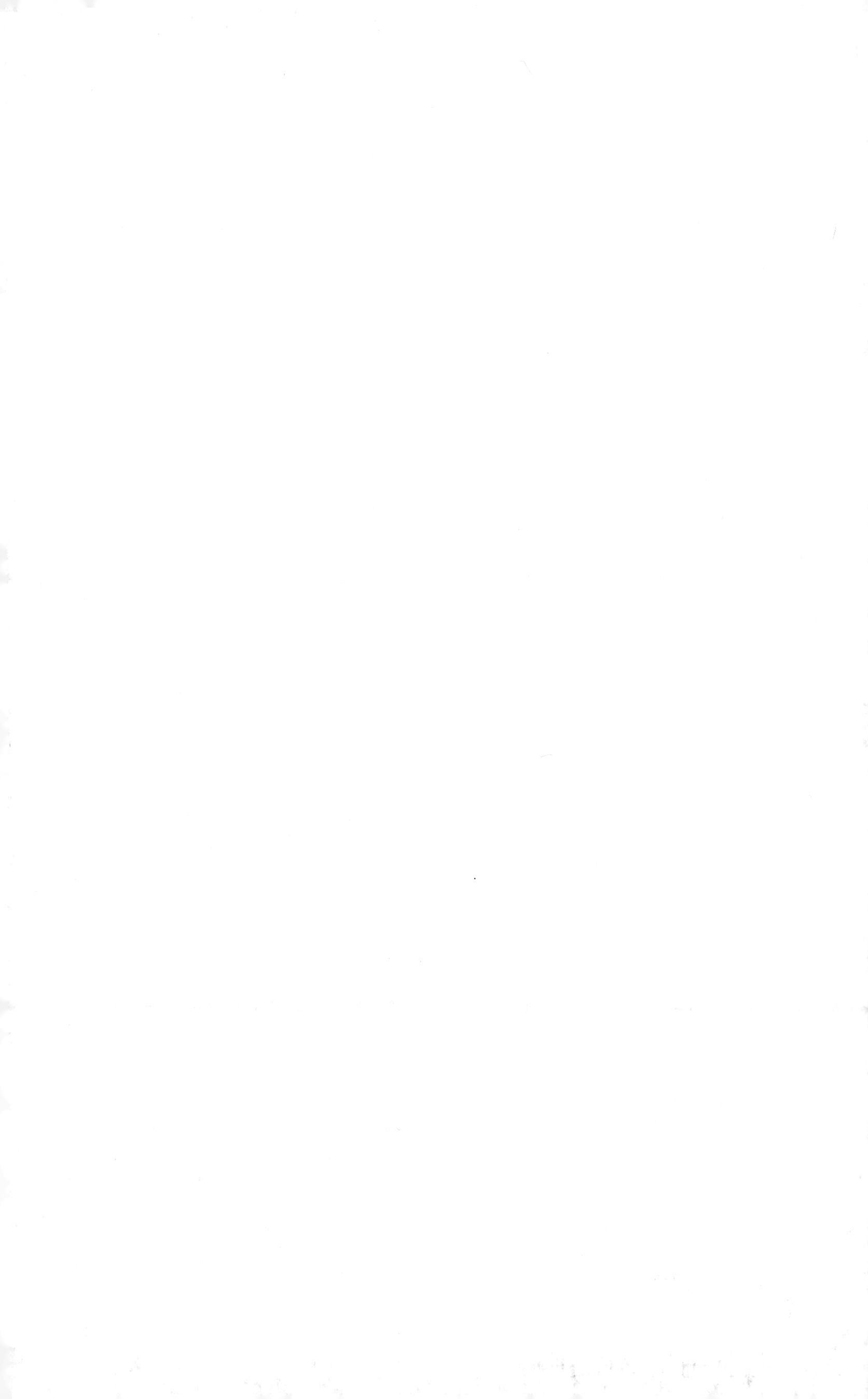